SOOTH

STAY OUT OF THE HOSPITAL

ANGELA LAWS

authorHOUSE®

AuthorHouse™
1663 Liberty Drive
Bloomington, IN 47403
www.authorhouse.com
Phone: 1 (800) 839-8640

Published by AuthorHouse 04/11/2016

ISBN: 978-1-5049-8280-1 (sc)
ISBN: 978-1-5049-8281-8 (e)

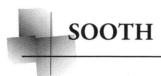 **SOOTH**

PLAN OF SUCCESS

Making sure you chart your Progress

People who regularly chart their blood pressure and sugar levels have a better understanding of how their body is working with medications prescribed by your doctor. Sometimes if you'r blood pressure stays high for a long period of time, it may mean the medication is not working. This means seeing your doctor, and maybe changing the medication your taking or the amount of the medication your taking.

Write Your Doctor's Appointments Down.

Writing your appointments down helps you to remember when you saw the doctor last, and when the next scheduled appointment is. This is very important information for your primary doctor, other doctors you may see. This can better your treatment by all doctors knowing your plan of care.

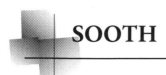 **SOOTH**

Stay out of the Hospital

Know your symptoms

There are many triggers that can
  Cause people to have negative
    Symptoms.
Are you eating more/less food than normal?

Do you feel that sometimes you hear or see
Things that others don't?

Are you seeing things/people no
One besides you can see?

Have you been sad for a long period of time?

Do you have thoughts of hurting yourself or others?
  If you are call 911

SOOTH

Take your medications

Know what medications your
   taking.
Ask your doctor to explain your
   medications to you.

Ask your doctor why you are on
   these medications.

Ask how often to take your
   Medications.

Ask if you need to eat with the
   Medication.

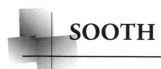

SOOTH

PLAN OF SUCCESS

Medication List:	What is Med For?

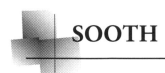 # SOOTH

PLAN OF SUCCESS

Dossage	Doctor

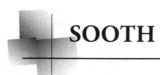

SOOTH

PLAN OF SUCCESS

Medication List:	What is Med For?

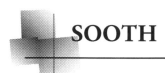 **SOOTH**

PLAN OF SUCCESS

Dossage

Doctor

SOOTH

Stay out of the Hospital

Keeping your appointments can keep **You** out of the hospital.

Write down your appointment
dates.

Get a Ride to the appointments
three days before appointment

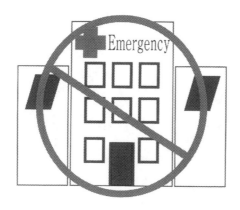

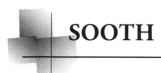 **SOOTH**

Stay out of the Hospital

Monday	Tuesday	Wednesday	Thursday	Friday	Saturday	Sunday

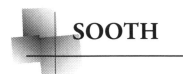

SOOTH

Stay out of the Hospital

Monday	Tuesday	Wednesday	Thursday	Friday	Saturday	Sunday

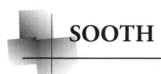# SOOTH

Stay out of the Hospital

Monday	Tuesday	Wednesday	Thursday	Friday	Saturday	Sunday

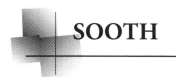

SOOTH

Stay out of the Hospital

Monday	Tuesday	Wednesday	Thursday	Friday	Saturday	Sunday

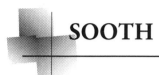

SOOTH

Stay out of the Hospital

Monday	Tuesday	Wednesday	Thursday	Friday	Saturday	Sunday

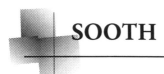

SOOTH

Stay out of the Hospital

Monday	Tuesday	Wednesday	Thursday	Friday	Saturday	Sunday

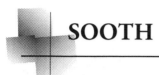

SOOTH

Stay out of the Hospital

Monday	Tuesday	Wednesday	Thursday	Friday	Saturday	Sunday

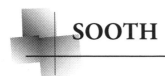

SOOTH

Stay out of the Hospital

Monday	Tuesday	Wednesday	Thursday	Friday	Saturday	Sunday

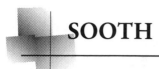

SOOTH

Stay out of the Hospital

Monday	Tuesday	Wednesday	Thursday	Friday	Saturday	Sunday

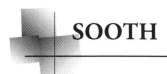

SOOTH

Stay out of the Hospital

Monday	Tuesday	Wednesday	Thursday	Friday	Saturday	Sunday

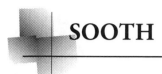

SOOTH

Stay out of the Hospital

Monday	Tuesday	Wednesday	Thursday	Friday	Saturday	Sunday

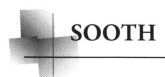

SOOTH

Stay out of the Hospital

Monday	Tuesday	Wednesday	Thursday	Friday	Saturday	Sunday

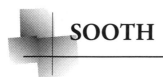

SOOTH

Stay out of the Hospital

Know your levels and weight

Diabetes:

Check your sugar daily before
and after meals.

Congestive Heart Failure:

Weigh yourself every morning.

High Blood Pressure:

Check your blood pressure
Daily.

Pneumonia:

Take all antibiotics

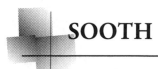 **SOOTH**

PLAN OF SUCCESS

Date	Time	Levels/amount

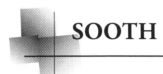 **SOOTH**

PLAN OF SUCCESS

Date	Time	Levels/amount

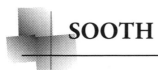

SOOTH

PLAN OF SUCCESS

Date	Time	Levels/amount

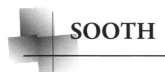

SOOTH

PLAN OF SUCCESS

Date	Time	Levels/amount

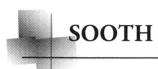

SOOTH

PLAN OF SUCCESS

Date	Time	Levels/amount

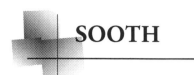 **SOOTH**

PLAN OF SUCCESS

Date	Time	Levels/amount

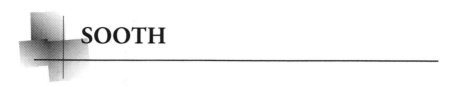

SOOTH

Stay out of the Hospital

NOTES

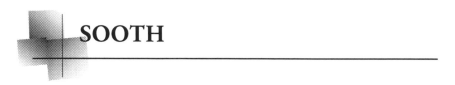

SOOTH

Stay out of the Hospital

NOTES

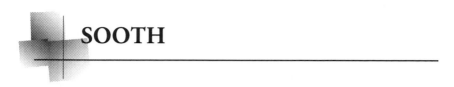

SOOTH

Stay out of the Hospital

NOTES

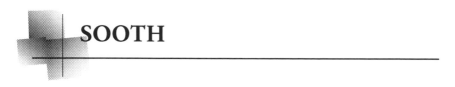

SOOTH

Stay out of the Hospital

NOTES

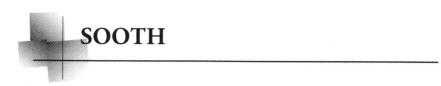

SOOTH

Stay out of the Hospital

NOTES

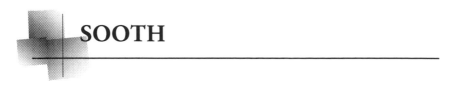

SOOTH

Stay out of the Hospital

NOTES

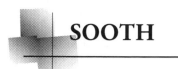

SOOTH

Stay out of the Hospital

NOTES

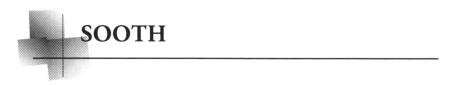

SOOTH

Stay out of the Hospital

NOTES

Printed in the United States
By Bookmasters